CHILDHOOD DISEASE

Understanding Childhood Disease, its Prevention & Reversal with a Plant Based Diet

The Medicine On Your Plate – Vol 5

By John Hodges & Ted Gif

www.viddapublishing.com

This edition published by
VIDDA Publishing Ltd in 2015. www.viddapublishing.com
Copyright © VIDDA Publishing Ltd 2015

While the author has made all reasonable efforts to ensure that the information contained in this book is accurate and up to date at the time of publication, anyone reading this book should note the following important points:-

Medical and pharmaceutical knowledge are constantly changing and the author and the publisher cannot and do not guarantee the accuracy or appropriateness of the contents of this book;

In any event, this book is not intended to be, and should not be relied upon, as a substitute for appropriate, tailored professional advice. Both the author and the publisher strongly recommend that a doctor or other healthcare professional is consulted before embarking on major dietary changes;

For the reasons set out above, and to the fullest extent permitted by law, the author and publisher: (i) cannot and do not accept any legal duty of care or responsibility in relation to the accuracy or appropriateness of the contents of this book, even where expressed as 'advice' or using other words to this effect; and (ii) disclaim any liability, loss, damage or risk that may be claimed or incurred as a consequence - directly or indirectly - of the use and/or application of any of the contents of this book.

Cover design by John Hodges.

VIDDA Publishing BOOK SHELF:
www.viddapublishing.com/books.html

Have you thought about self-publishing via Amazon Kindle? If so to make the process easier and more productive, I highly recommend this software to help you on your way.

KBookPromotion: bit.ly/KBookPromotion

Your FREE Gift

Thank you for purchasing this book. To show our appreciation we would like to offer you a copy of our FREE recipe book "BRING LIFE TO YOUR FOOD". To download, visit our website: **www.viddapublishing.com**.

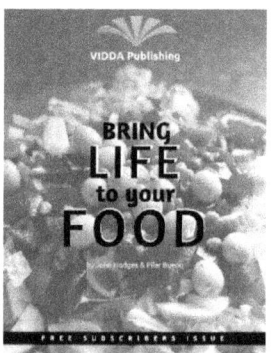

If you're interested in Health, Nutrition, Green and / or Cruelty-Free products please visit our Websites and online **VIDDA Health Stores** (US: bit.ly/VIDDAstore & UK: bit.ly/VIDDAstoreUK).

www.viddapublishing.com

www.sirtfood.com

www.themedicineonyourplate.com

www.greenupyourlife.org

www.ecologizatuvida.com

Table of Content

Introduction: Diet and Disease Prevention

It is taken as a given that a modicum of education and awareness around *"food"* in its widest possible sense is necessary if the metabolism is to remain healthy. For many people the reasons for adopting a Plant Based Diet (PBD) centre on notions of, looking after the environment, animal rights, the unnatural nature of intensive farming and the potential for animal-borne diseases such as BSE. The reasons to adopt a PBD range from the practical to the emotional to the medicinally necessary. The nutritional aspects of a PBD are not irrelevant; they are an intrinsic foundation and reason to make the decision in the first place. With particular reference to preventable and childhood disease, It is these nutritional aspects that will form the subject matter of this book. In its entirety this series of books presents evidence that a PBD (that is a balanced diet which contains no animal products whatsoever) plays a vital role in preventing metabolic disease. Many of these diseases such as Type-2 diabetes and Cardio Vascular Disease (CVD) express a personal, financial and community cost which can be largely avoided by eating a PBD. In other words, by making a choice to eat such a diet you are alleviating a financial pressure on health care provision and potentially facilitating longer life and acknowledging the issues mentioned above. This final book is, in essence, an overview of why it is possible to make these assertions. This volume begins with an explanation of what is meant by a plant based diet and from there we will be dealing with the principle myths concerning a vegan and vegetarian and diet. The remaining chapters will present the overall case for adopting a PBD with particular reference to preventable and childhood disease. The five books presented in this set are in a very real sense merely the tip of a tip of a very large iceberg. As usual, the reader is encouraged to follow up on the hyperlinks presented.

Chapter 1:
What is a Plant based Diet?

It is a fact that non-communicable disease (NCD) is a bigger global killer than a communicable disease. In addition, the proportion of those killed by NCD is steadily rising. For example, according to the World Health Organisation (WHO), the total global percentage of persons killed by NCD rose from 60% in the year 2000 to almost 70% in 2012. Furthermore, as the current situation stands, there is no need to suppose that this upward trend will cease. The big four global NCD killers are CVD, cancer, diabetes and lung / bronchial cancer. The single biggest killer is CVD which kills approximately 20 million persons annually. In the UK CVD, stroke, cancer as well lung and the liver disease kill over 150,000 people every year and it is estimated that about a fifth of these deaths is preventable. For example, research consistently shows that those who follow a PBD have lower blood pressure, lower levels of LDL cholesterol (the form you don't want) and so a putative lower incidence of CVD and related conditions can be inferred. In other words, the risk of acquiring a disease as a result of a bad diet is reduced. A principle driver behind this notion is the reality that a PBD contains more fibre, folates, vitamins and minerals, phytochemicals (including flavonoids and anti-oxidants) all of which are directly connected with producing lower levels of LDL as compared to omnivorous diets. In addition, a PBD diet based on fresh, unprocessed foods that you have prepared yourself on balance contains more nutrients across the board than any other eating pattern you may choose to adopt.

The *"crushing diabetes"* book imparted the difference between type-1 and type-2 diabetes and inculcates that the latter is largely preventable by dietary means. Type-two diabetes accounts for some 90% of all cases and is, in essence, a direct symptom of the global obesity epidemic which was additionally alluded to in the *"SIRT FOOD"* book. Once again it is the majority world which bears the brunt of these figures with about 75% of all 40 million deaths from NCD occurring in the global south. Interestingly, the proportion of actual deaths from NCD is greater in high-income countries than in low-income countries. Furthermore, the overwhelming majority of deaths in the "rich" world occur over the age of 70 but in the majority world, most deaths occur under the age of 15. If you think about it, the final two assertions indicate the disgraceful status of health care which exists for the majority of people on the planet. The evidence that the western diet and associated lifestyle are directly implicated in the incidence of obesity, diabetes, CVD, cancer and even arthritis, is so overwhelming that it can almost be said to be bordering on scientific truth. All over the world the virtues of a plant based diet as a form of nutritional therapy are increasingly apparent. A PBD is a diet which:

- Removes all animal (including fish and chicken!), dairy products (including eggs)

- Removes all refined and processed foodstuffs

- Embraces the eating of the whole plant and grain foods and their derivatives.

For our purposes, we are looking at a PBD which is as free from processed and refined foods. If you are eating *"junk"* vegetarian food it's still a junk food diet and you will still be prone to the negative health consequences of such a diet. Nutritional therapy is in the widest possible sense is a more scientific term for the phrase *"eating a balanced diet"*. Both are concerned with ensuring that the body receives all the essential compounds it needs for optimal or homeostatic metabolism. One clear cut difference lays with the use of the word *"therapy"*, if a child (or anyone else for that matter), is affected by a disease or life threatening condition, then the diet is concerned with eating foods that may boost the ability of the body to deal with the ailment. Nutritional therapy seeks to establish whether a particular diet can redress any nutritional imbalance and so strengthen the response to a given illness or disease whilst continuing to ensure physiological and emotional well-being. Overall, research consistently shows that a PBD diet is affordable, provided the individual educates themselves as to what it is to actually be a *"vegetarian"* or *"vegan"* and takes control of their eating habits. In normal parlance this means buying a cookbook, using it, learning the food groups and gaining a grounding of what actually happens to them when they are eaten. As we shall see in chapter two self-educating will enable the reader to dispel the tired myths concerning the virtues of a PBD.

Overall a PBD has demonstrable and almost immediate benefits on all of the negative health conditions either indicated or discussed throughout this set of books. The reader need only follow up on the hyperlinks and sources presented to appreciate this; you will find an enormous amount of information on the role of diet in effective health care. Furthermore, there are literally thousands (if not more) examples of individuals who have gone to their doctor or hospital with any one (or more) of these conditions. These individuals have been told to basically change their dietary ways and embrace a Mediterranean or PBD and have then enjoyed health benefits which have presented themselves within weeks. The reason is simple, a balanced PBD will by definition enable a person to eat foods which are packed with all the nutrients the body needs for healthy metabolism.

Nobody is perfect in this sphere but a PBD means eating fresh fruit and vegetables, pulses, grains, nuts and seeds with a minimum of additional fat, salt, preservatives or other synthetic (human-made) ingredients. The individual molecules which are synthesised (by condensation polymerization) into proteins are but one example of the benefits of eating a PBD diet.

Aside from being the building blocks for proteins, amino acids help to regulate the activity of the hormones insulin and glucagon. Hence the type of protein that is ingested through feeding has the potential to influence the activity of both chemical messengers. It is known that plant-derived proteins tend to stimulate the production of glucagon in preference to insulin. Aside from stimulating the body to convert glucose into glycogen, glucagon also inhibits the activity of enzymes which are known to promote the formation of fats. This is important because a PBD which is high in fibre and low in saturated fats amplifies this effect, further inhibiting the production of insulin. In addition, there is ample evidence which suggests a vegan diet reduces the risk of developing the cancers associated with the western diet. This was discussed in the *"crushing cancer"* Book and in terms of colorectal cancer, there is definite evidence that eating excessive amounts of red meat (over 90g) per day increases the risk of developing this form of cancer. In short eating a full PBD in conjunction with regular exercise has proven health benefits across the board. Whether these benefits extend to a causative link to a particular disease is another matter, never the less, science tells us that an association exists and therefore opportunity to reduce risk present itself. In terms of CVD lifestyle changes in chronically overweight and obese persons are known reduce the incidence of atherosclerosis as compared to control groups. This is another way of saying that if a person is diagnosed with a CVD where diet is implicated as a cause, the condition can be potentially reversed. Such an assertion can be applied to CVD in general as well as stenosis (narrowing of any blood vessel), stroke and chronically high blood pressure in particular. Overall the incidence of CVD and associated conditions can be reduced by adopting a balanced PBD. Furthermore, researchers in the field of CVD impart that the single biggest preventative measure (aside from ditching tobacco smoking) that a person can adopt is to cut down on eating red meat.

One of my core arguments has always been that it doesn't matter what you think or believe, it is down to a very large extent what the science reveals. I have had to change my mind or alter my view more times than I care to remember. Surely, a healthy mindset to have if you want to be well rounded informed and cognizant human being.

The same is true in the field of diet and nutrition such that there is now overwhelming evidence which suggests that a PBD can facilitate the prevention and even roll back the biological impacts and symptoms of the biggest killers in the Western World. A huge foundation for this assertion is that plants contain in their entirety more of the phytochemicals (which include flavonoids and anti-oxidants) which the body requires for healthy nutrition and a stable metabolism. As was explained in the *"crushing arthritis"* and other books, the phytochemicals are a family of individual molecules numbering at least in the several thousand and the biochemical basis for their efficacy continues to be revealed. Although physicians who operated thousands of years ago would not have used such scientific language, they knew which plants and herbs helped with particular ailments and / or injuries. In the 21st century, we know many of the active compounds used in the treatment of disease are in fact derived from plants. The use of plant based compounds to treat disease is in the widest possible sense is termed phytotherapy (from the word phytochemical). Put simply animal foods do not contain as many phytochemicals as plants and so clearly, eating more plants means you are ingesting more of these chemicals. There is no such thing as a one-size fits all PBD and as such you will need to experiment and evaluate what is best for your own circumstances. Once again, if you have been *"told"* to dump the western diet and adopt a PBD then you will need to follow the advice of the professionals in the field. For example, you may be prescribed a diet low in sodium and potassium to reduce your blood pressure, which may be required if you have a family history of stroke, hypertension or CVD in general. It must be stressed that a PBD will not categorically prevent any NCD; it will, however, greatly reduce the risk of developing such a condition. In short, a wide and well-balanced PBD contains all of the nutrients that the body requires through all stages of life. As the next chapter will indicate education and awareness of what is meant by nutrition is absolutely essential.

Chapter 2:
Dispelling the Myths

Adopting a PBD diet does not mean simply removing meat, fish and dairy products from the diet and just doubling up on the fruits and vegetables you would eat normally. It means understanding some basic food and nutrition science and eating as wide a possible range of foods which are not derived from animals. It is important to realise that a PBD is not some dietary fad which resides in the town of Quackville, it is characterised by what it includes and as an individual you are encouraged to eat as many different plant foods as possible. In other words, if you like chips, you don't have to give them up, you just buy some potatoes and learn how to make your own. My personal preference is sautéed potatoes with, sliced onion, garlic, marjoram, rosemary and a hint of thyme. Preparation time is about 10 minutes and cooking time about 30, a little less if you par boil. The point is there is no great secret to eating well on a PBD. However, we do need to clearly define some key terms:

- A vegan diet excludes all animal products and should never be undertaken without educating yourself and / or seeking nutritional advice.

- A vegetarian / lacto-ovo diet excludes all meat and seafood but does include dairy products.

- A Lacto vegetarian excludes eggs, meat (including poultry) but does include milk products.

- An Ovo-vegetarian is a diet which excludes all animal, seafood and dairy products except eggs.

- A Mediterranean diet is essentially a vegetarian diet with small and measured amounts of fish, poultry, red meat and dairy products.

- Whole food PBD is where plant foods are eaten with the minimum of preparation. In particular the eating of whole fruits, vegetables, nuts and seeds. Animal products and fats are severely restricted with this diet.

Now, these definitions do not require an either, or approach and you should seek to explore which food groups suit you best. It goes without saying that if you are eating food as a preventative measure for disease or you are in any kind recovery or remission the advice of a trained nutritionist, dietician and / or doctor should be sought. Overall, the goal of the diet is to improve your health and should not be viewed as a chore or something that is difficult or undesirable. In other words, you have to want to make these lifestyle and dietary changes. Overall, the wider the range of foods you eat the greater are the levels of fibre, vitamins, minerals and phytochemicals (including flavonoids and carotenoids), as compared to a western or omnivorous diet. In and of itself this has to be desirable! So, let us picture the scene, you have been invited to a dinner party or equivalent and you have said *"no animals for me"*, what are arguments extolling the folly of your position might you encounter? In no particular order let us have a look at the most likely *"you what"* comments:

1. YOU WON'T GET ENOUGH PROTEIN: This is perhaps the biggest source of disinformation concerning the virtues of a PBD. It is also not true, simply because all plant foods contain proteins and provided you are eating a wide and varied whole food and PBD your metabolism will be able to digest all the proteins it needs. In other

words, it is absolutely possible for a person eating a PBD to obtain all the essential amino acids they need for healthy metabolism. The products of this digestion, the amino acids, will then be re-synthesised into the proteins your body needs for its metabolism. In other words, you do not need to eat meat, fish or dairy products to obtain all the proteins you need. All proteins are made from the same amino acids and so provided the plant foods contain those amino acids there will be no issues here. You will need to plenty of pulses, nuts, brown rice, seeds and perhaps look at replacing dairy milk with almond milk.

2. A PBD WILL BREAK THE BANK AND BE TOO TIME CONSUMING: Here's an idea that may convince you that the expense of a PBD is all down to perspective, try keeping a food diary for a week. Record the expense of what you eat *"normally"* and then for the next follow a PBD diet and then put the difference in the jar marked *"holiday"*. I invite you to comment and tell me that all things being equal that a PBD is more expensive than your normal diet. You will need to avoid processed, packaged and convenience food, and use that all important cookbook. As for the time issue, well, guess what? Cooking does take more time than throwing a ready meal in the oven; however, as with all worthwhile pursuits, the benefits will more than outweigh any extra time cooking takes. Also once you get stuck into the kitchen you'll find that your portion sizes will adapt to your needs and once you start getting into the habit of making a bit more for lunch the next day, that holiday jar will fill up with sheckles very quickly indeed.

3. YOUR APPETITE WILL NEVER BE SATISFIED: Well as an unapologetic foodie, I can say this is utter nonsense. If you feel constantly hungry its either that your PBD is not

balanced enough, namely not enough fibre, slow release carbohydrates, fats or proteins, or something else is wrong. As has been (I hope) been made abundantly clear you are choosing to adopt a PBD and that means you need to experiment with different recipes. Remember adopting a PBD is also all about educating yourself and there are no short cuts in this endeavour, so you need to get to grips with what is going on with your metabolism. For example, fibre (or dietary roughage) is essentially indigestible (along with cellulose), but it does keep the intestines feeling full. It also helps the body to properly regulate blood glucose levels, which help prevent cravings. Fresh foods are generally slower to digest than processed foods, but yes we all like a little snack, I know I do like I said I'm a foodie. So get some nuts and raisins in a bowl and see for yourself.

4. A PBD IS BORING AND THE FOOD IS TASTELESS: Sorry, but this all down to perception, speaking personally, I hate sprouts, turnip and can only tolerate sweet potatoes in soups, stews or broths and nothing on this Earth is going to change that fact. The reason is texture and the taste literally makes me want to gag, other people have the same response to mushrooms and carrots and there are plenty of people who are vegetarian or vegan because they cannot abide the taste of meat or fish. As for the notion that a PBD is unattractive, well that's down to getting stuck into cooking and learning about presentation and colour. It has been written throughout these volumes that you will need to get stuck in the kitchen, there is no short cut; you will need to get yourself a decent no nonsense cookbook as was described in the "SIRT FOOD" book. Such a proposition should be something to look forward to; if it's not then I would

argue that you need to change your attitude! There are literally hundreds of different plants, nuts grains, pulses and the like to discover and you need to dive in, so off you go.

5. YOU WILL FEEL LETHARGIC AND WITHOUT ENERGY: Again, if you're feeling tired it's probably not the diet and if after visiting your doctor they say it is, then you are doing it wrong. The one area of a PBD that you do need to be on top of is the ingestion of vitamin B12 and Iron. Vitamin B12 is essential for the production of blood cells and helps regulate the rate of cell division (mitosis). It is produced by bacteria as part of their metabolism and so is not produced by plants or animals. A PBD can more than adequately meet the metabolic need for iron from foods such as spinach, pulses, lentils and cashew nuts, to name but a few. To counter this particular argument you can extol the virtues of a balanced diet by saying something like, *"ok fair point, but I also eat plenty of tomatoes, broccoli and citrus fruits"*. These foods all contain vitamin C (ascorbic acid) which amongst its other benefits is known to aid in the absorption of iron. As for vitamin B12 well, I've just checked the ingredients on a jar of marmite and guess what it's loaded with this highly essential vitamin! Ok so let's say you're a *"hater"* of this most wonderful spread, well there are other yeast based spreads, which are more palatable. Aside from marmite or equivalent spread then your best course of action are fortified foodstuffs or under the instruction of a trained professional a dietary supplement.

There are plenty more arguments and counter arguments so at the end of the day it's up to you. It must be realised that a PBD is not some sort of panacea or *"get out of jail free"* card toward obtaining a disease free life because it isn't. I have had to field the above comments when I said I wanted to be vegetarian because I disagreed with factory farming. I was called everything from *"a wimpy wet drip"* to a *"poncy trendy leftie"* and that was just my family! In addition, some members of my social circle at the time were incredulous to the point of mortification. If you are going to adopt a PBD you have to want to do it and irrespective of your motivations don't let anyone tell you that there is somehow *"something wrong"* with such an undertaking. It cannot be understated that a proper balanced PBD is going to require some changes to your lifestyle but these changes must be set against the long-term health benefits of adopting the diet, surely a core reason for taking control of your eating habits in the first place.

There are all sorts of reasons for adopting a PBD or at least cutting down on the foods which fall into the box ticked *"western diet"*. There are sound environmental reasons for not eating factory farmed meat but those same arguments can also be applied to processed vegetarian foods. Overall, all that is being said is that there are demonstrable nutritional benefits to a PBD and wholefood diet. Generally speaking, those who follow a PBD have a lower risk of CVD, Type-2 diabetes, obesity and some types of cancer. A PBD also appears to allow the body to ingest in abundance the intake of vitamins, minerals and phytochemicals instead of the substances implicated in the above diseases.

Chapter 3:
Diet, Breast-Feeding and Disease

The risk of developing any kind of dietary related condition will vary according to many variables but what we can say is that good nutrition begins in the womb. This means that from a dietary perspective preventative steps can be taken at the outset of pregnancy. In the early stages of life (including as a foetus), a balanced metabolism is essential. For example, both delayed and excessive weight gain have been shown to be linked to chronic CVD, stroke as well as both forms of diabetes. Other studies suggest that shorter children who grow too quickly are at an increased risk of stroke and childhood cancers. Overall, there is a fair body of research which indicates that the growth of children who at a PBD is more regular and staged than for an omnivorous diet and that there is no difference in height by the end of adolescence. The point is that too rapid growth has been implicated in an increased risk of disease in later life. This google search reveals the degree of primary research on the subject followed by the corpus of secondary knowledge, so feel free to dive in!

In the frame of childhood disease, it is essential to inculcate that the majority of child deaths still occur in the global South. The figures are particularly disgusting for infant mortality, according to the WHO approximately 7 million children died before their fifth birthday in 2012. Over 99% of these lives were snuffed out by largely preventable diseases. Arguably the exception is malaria which accounts for 15% of the total infant mortality in sub-Saharan Africa. I write arguably because the incidence of malaria can be reduced by providing adequate health care for the regions where it occurs. Clearly, such provision is not at the forefront of the minds of our so-called leaders. If it were I would not be seeing calls for funding from organisations such as UNICEF. The biggest child killers in the global south are premature birth, pneumonia, strangulation and asphyxiation at birth and diarrhoeal diseases such as cholera and amoebic dysentery. Approximately 45% of all infant deaths occur within 28 days of Birth and the single biggest killer accounting for 35% of the figures was in 2012 premature birth. All of this occurring against a backdrop where child mortality rates are actually falling but malnutrition contributes to almost half of all deaths and so at least 3.5 million children die unnecessarily every year because they do not have enough to eat. I'm willing to bet that communities where such infant mortality occurs (where ever they are), would love to have the individual choices that can be exercised here in the developed world.

OK returning to the Northern Hemisphere! Clearly, pregnancy is not the time to start experimenting with the diet. As such the advice of a trained medical professional on all dietary and nutritional requirements should be sought as a matter of course. Hence, this chapter will assume that a PBD diet is the norm and that the pregnant woman is well versed in the virtues of adopting it. Overall, a well-planned and organised PBD will more than meet the nutritional needs of the pregnant woman and gestating foetus. What can be clearly stated is that a pregnant woman does need to gain some weight but this gain will not result in the negative health consequences of the justifiably savaged *"western diet"*. For all the wrong reasons this diet replete with all its nutritional deficits exemplifies that *"you are what you eat"*, meaning that our diet to a very large extent determines our health, well-being, growth and development. For example the WHO presents evidence which fortifies the idea that breastfeeding may reduce the future risk of developing obesity and NCD disease in general. In addition, the breast milk formulas do not offer the same level of health protection as the breast milk. For example the differences in fatty acid composition have been well documented and are still the subject of on-going research. In addition (despite the protestations of the manufacturers) the negative impacts of breast milk formula are well documented and associated with conditions such as type-1 diabetes and the cancers generally associated with adolescence.

For example, essential fatty acids are known to have a whole range of developmental roles. Most of the individual molecules or family they are part of having a multi-functional role in metabolism, growth and development. For example DocosaHexaenoic Acid (DHA $C_{22}H_{32}O_2$) is a long chain fatty acid essential (amongst other roles) for the development of the brain and eyes. DHA is not produced directly by the body; it is derived from omega 3 oils with the main non-plant source of this substance being oily and / or cold water fish. In a PBD the principal dietary source is olive oil as well as various nuts and seeds especially flaxseed which can be incorporated into, cereals, bread, soups and salads. However, these sources also contain omega 6 oils which are known to inhibit the conversion of omega 3 oils to substances such as DHA. Overall the advice is to maximise all opportunities your ingestion of omega 3 oils whilst minimising that of omega 6 oils. In addition, dieticians recommend that a PBD diet during pregnancy must contain linolenic acid, which is obtained from several plant based foodstuffs. Put simply linolenic acid is converted by our metabolism into DHA and other fatty acid compounds and so acts as an alternative food source to fish derived omega 3 oils. Linolenic acid has utility in the treatment of Arthritis, Multiple Sclerosis, lupus, diabetes and Chrons disease. In other words, the substance is potentially important for treating auto-immune disease.

Almost all infants are breastfed for the first few months of their lives but after this time the numbers begin to steadily fall and according to researchers in the US, the rate of decline is higher for women who are non-vegetarian. Even during breastfeeding rates appear to be higher for vegan and vegetarian women as compared to omnivorous mothers. For example, rates of up to 95% have been recorded for vegan women, 90% for vegetarian women, but in the case of omnivorous women, rates can drop to as low as 65%. Overall, such findings give a strong indication that women following a PBD are more likely to breastfeed their infants and for a longer period of time than those who are omnivores. Hence if we adhere to the notion that "breast is best" then we can infer that a PBD during pregnancy is no less associated with the birth of a healthy child than with an omnivorous diet and that during weaning vegan and vegetarian mothers breastfeed their infants for a longer time.

Aside from the emotional, psychological and bonding aspects the nutritional benefits of breastfeeding are clear and present. Overall in the northern hemisphere children who are not breastfed are more prone to disease across the board and according to researchers more likely die before their first birthday. In addition, breastfeeding has been clearly associated with a reduced incidence of obesity, both forms of diabetes, Sudden Infant Death Syndrome (SIDS) and leukaemia. In addition, there are well documented negative health impacts for mothers themselves who do not breastfeed their babies. In other words, breastfeeding is likely an evolutionary mechanism by which mother and child are given the best possible chance of survival. For me, that is reason enough to encourage breastfeeding for as long as it is beneficial to the infant and mother to do so. Breastfeeding is by far the most effective way for an infant to obtain all the crucial compounds needed for his or her metabolism, this is especially true up to 6 months old. Little wonder that The American College of Obstetricians and Gynaecologists (ACOG) recommends 6 months of total feeding with breast milk, a position endorsed by equivalent organisations in the US and Europe. The WHO further recommends that breastfeeding ought to be an option up until the second birthday of the child. With that kind of heavyweight scientific backing, it is quite staggering that the figures of uptake for the U.S, the UK (although the number is rising) as compared to significant numbers of Eurasian countries, fall so short of this six-month guideline.

Aside from the nutritional benefits the main principle reason why *"breast is best"* is down to the unique immune system boosting properties of the breast milk. During pregnancy cells from the bronchial network (the lungs) and from the intestines are transported by the circulatory system to the breasts when they start producing milk. Once there the milk becomes laden with the same factors which cause immunity in the mother, by definition formula milk cannot provide this level of protection. For example, specialist carbohydrates called oligosaccharides (carbohydrates composed of between two and twenty monomer molecules) are known to prevent various respiratory pathogens from infecting the growing baby. Similarly, a class of biological molecules called glycoproteins (a protein with at least one carbohydrate molecule attached) prevent intestinal pathogens from expressing themselves. The list of benefits is as complex as it is comprehensive and the reader should follow up on any strands of this writing as they see fit. The calcium content of breast milk is not affected by adopting a vegan balanced PBD, so by definition, it won't be affected by a vegetarian or Mediterranean diet either. Once the first six months of life are passed it will probably be opportune to begin introducing solid foods (weaning). Concurrently, there is no reason not to begin introducing the complete availability whole and plant based foods. In later life, it is up to the parents to discuss with their children the virtues of a PBD and whether or not they should partake of a Mediterranean diet, remember it is a lifestyle choice and not an imposition.

Right, lecture over, back to Calcium! The dietary levels of this essential mineral must be monitored so that healthy ossification (bone formation) occurs. Calcium is also essential for rapid blood clotting and the effective function of the nervous system because it facilitates the transmission of electrical impulses inside both the cardiac (heart) muscles and musculoskeletal system. Foods which are rich sources of calcium are kale, cabbage and leafy green (collard) vegetables in general. Helpfully, these vegetables are also concentrated sources of additional essential vitamins and minerals. After six months age, the constituents of the diet become progressively more important. For instance, human breast milk contains all of the zinc an infant needs up to about age 7 months, after which time zinc must come from the diet. Zinc functions by boosting the immune system and promoting rapid healing of cuts and abrasions. The plant based sources of zinc are wide and varied, but it must be stated that plants do not contain as much zinc as they do other trace minerals. However, herbs such as basil and thyme can be added as they both contain relatively high concentrations of zinc. Good food sources of zinc include pulses, grains and asparagus.

In the interests of balance, the only credible nutritional arguments concerning a PBD are the potential risk of becoming deficient in vitamin B12 and Iron. However, it can also be supposed that the western diet in its entirety is so lacking in nutrients that a stones and glass houses scenario may well present itself. However, the point remains that during pregnancy the woman is *"eating for two"* and all nutrients play a vital role in maintaining the health of both expectant mother and her developing foetus. The same can be said for other vitamin and mineral deficiencies. A deficiency of vitamin D during pregnancy is common in the northern hemisphere and as such deficiency in newborn infants irrespective of the diet is not uncommon. Whilst concrete data on comparing the weight of infants born to mothers who followed a PBD as compared to those who did not is somewhat sparse, there is no evidence of a discrepancy as indicated by the few epidemiological studies on the subject. In fact, the Rowan paper referenced below suggests that babies born to mothers following a PBD had the highest average birth weights and none had low birth weights as compared omnivorous mothers. This is merely an indicator and no causative link between birth weight and diet is being suggested.

Without any scaremongering or hysteria, if it is true that eating meat (in particular red meat) can have undesirable health impacts on adults and teenagers, then the same must be true of a gestating foetus and mother. Without a doubt, there are plenty of studies which present associations of negative health conditions with eating animal foods. For example, there have been suggested links between the cessation of breastfeeding within the six-month guideline and the onset of type-one diabetes. Such that for infants fed on cow's milk at three months the risk of this form of diabetes is higher than infants who are fed for three months or longer. Again such findings do not present a causative link, they suggest if not directly imply that after pregnancy breastfeeding should be the norm for at least the recommended six months of life.

Chapter 4:
Children and a PBD

The uptake of unhealthy and dietary and lifestyle choices in our formative and adolescent years have a very real potential to traverse into serious and chronic negative biological conditions in adult life. In other words, risk factors ranging from smoking to diet are directly associated (if not implicated) to adult CVD, Diabetes, hypertension and cancer, to name a few of the preventable conditions. In addition once a preventable disease has taken hold it is much more difficult to deal with, clearly, then, prevention is better than cure. In other words, the risk factors associated with childhood diseases are more than able to cross into adult life. Hence if children can be encouraged to adopt more healthy dietary and lifestyle choices they are significantly more likely to enjoy longer periods of health and vitality in adulthood. Children and young people can be notoriously fussy eaters and this can (and likely will) be exacerbated by the onset of any disease. In turn, fussiness will be further augmented by any emotional trauma which is certain to be intrinsic to diagnoses of a disease. Such stresses in the formative years are likely to augment any feelings of *"losing control"* that a young person may have. The ability to choose what is eaten as well when, where and how or even with whom it is eaten could become an area that the child can *"control"* and so the advice from professionals in the field is to talk openly with your child and show flexibility in all areas connected to diet and nutrition but within well-established boundaries. Parents are also advised to educate themselves as much as possible about the metabolic processes affected by the disease.

There is no nutritional reason why a teenager or younger person should be discouraged from adopting a PBD. The myths alluded to in chapter two apply just as much to those of us who are starting out in life as they do to the rest of us. As has been made abundantly clear throughout these 5 volumes a PBD is directly associated with a lower risk of developing several serious (and /or potentially so) preventable diseases as compared to an animal based diet. Hence it is entirely possible for children and young people to adopt a PBD and be perfectly healthy as long as the diet is wide-ranging and balanced. For young people the metabolic demands of the body are different for adults as they are for the elderly and this reality must be factored into the dietary regimen. This does not mean that you must eat raw carrots dipped in hummus at 08.00am every day and nothing else, it means that you must take control of what you are eating. If you are a parent of a child who has chosen to adopt a PBD and you are clueless about what that choice actually means, then guess what? The onus is on you to educate yourself and your child as view the choice as a positive development that is to be encouraged.

Young people need to pay particular attention to intakes of vitamins protein, iron, zinc, calcium in particular and other trace minerals as advised. Overall, the PBD must be tweaked to ensure that it contains more of all the essential food groups, minerals and vitamins. For example, iron deficiency is arguably the single biggest nutritional deficiency in young people and so foods which contain this mineral such as dark beans, cereal grains and cruciferous vegetables must form part of the diet, in balance with other essential nutritional requirements. In other words to adopt a PBD A young person will need to know what they are eating and where all of the active substance come from. Furthermore, it must be reiterated that we are all different and so will have varying requirements and that these requirements will vary with age and gender as well as the stage of adolescence. The essential point of the writing of this book is to make clear that medication is not necessarily the answer to a given set of conditions. This does not mean I am advocating a cessation of any therapy or course of treatment. What is being suggested is that the root cause of the complaint needs to be established. Any google search will bring forward real testimonials and stories where dietary changes were made and health conditions improved. The reason is not that the drugs themselves don't function more that they were unnecessary for the circumstances in hand.

For instance, the Huffington post article referenced below is but one example of a dietary cause of an autoimmune condition. In this case, inflammation caused by an allergy to gluten and the lactose contained within dairy products. At this juncture, it is important that I point out the very likely role that genetically modified organisms (GMO's) have on the rise in the numbers of people experiencing gluten intolerance (and other dietary complaints) in the US and other countries which have adopted GM technology since the 1990's. The reader is invited to watch this space for more damming evidence as to why this wholly dysfunctional technology of genetic modification of food needs to be dumped forthwith! Ok, so back to the task at hand. In this Huffington post story once the dietary cause of the disease was established the medication could be ceased and the patient was as healthy as her peers. Once again I am not slating the medical profession I am just saying that the underlying cause of the condition (whatever it is) must be established before very powerful prescription drugs are administered. Concurrently, it would seem logical to begin this process by looking at the diet. If you think about it, if a dietary element to the aetiology (cause) of any disease can be established then it seems reasonable to suppose that at the very least improving the diet can alleviate symptoms. Such dietary changes need to be combined with the uptake of some form of exercise and reducing stress levels. The last area may prove to be difficult if *"things are going on at home"* or if a crucial test or exam is on the horizon.

The role of "Big pharma" in the treatment of disease and the development of medicine was alluded to in the *"crushing cancer"* book and so it raises its ugly head again. In very simple terms this oligarchy exists to sell prescription and non-prescription drugs to treat disease. Hence if it can be established that a particular disease or set of diseases can be managed or treated without recourse to various pills, potions, powders as well injections and infusions thereof, then it will be against the interest of the oligarchy to promote it. After all, if you are getting to root cause of an illness and you establish that the cause of a particular condition is a food which causes inflammation, irritation or even allergy, then you don't need a prescription to treat it. The bottom line is that for preventable diseases, even where a genetic predisposition exists) there is likely to be a metabolic trigger which promotes the onset of the condition. Equally, the trigger could be an illness or polluting substance interfering with normal physiology. The point is that the diet should not be discounted or ignored; it should be fully integrated into establishing the cause of any disease.

Provided the PBD is balanced there is absolutely no impact on the growth and development of a child who is adopting or eating a PBD. It is also fair to say that if the western diet is undesirable for the metabolism of adults than it must be more so for the developing child. Concurrently, if healthy eating habits can be instilled at an early age then they will almost certainly carry on into adulthood. One tried and tested method of achieving such an eventuality is involving children in the shopping and cooking process. Children are naturally curious and will participate in all food related activities and will soon let you know if they don't like a particular food. Clearly, if they are turning down too many foods then this may be an indicator of an underlying issue. There is also plenty of evidence which demonstrates that aside from good dietary and weight outcomes, that a PBD garners fewer problems with digestion, food allergies and intolerances and even with that scourge of adolescence acne. However, a causative link between acne and diet has yet to be established. In addition, if a person has severe acne than the advice of a dermatologist or equivalent professional should be sought. Additionally, a fair degree of evidence exists which suggests that puberty (particularly in girls) begins earlier if the diet contains excessive amounts of hormones which disrupt the endocrine system of young children. Clearly, a guaranteed way to minimise this risk is to not eat foods which contain the by-products of intensive animal farming. All that is being suggested is that a PBD diet is certainly not undesirable, affordable and workable for the metabolism of young people and it may in time prove to have very real benefits.

Chapter 5:
Diet and Childhood Arthritis

Hundreds of millions of people the world over are affected by the onset of some form of the rheumatoid disease. We generally associate arthritis as a disease of ageing, I mean we all have elderly relatives who impart that their bones are stiff. I heard my now deceased grandmother say *"Och well, I'm 87 you know and I've just shrunk a bit, it disnae' matter"*, Well I guess at that age maybe it doesn't matter so much, however, the same is not true if you are at the opposite end of life. That is as the same grandmother used to say *"It's away sad wits happenin' tae the young yin's the day, just startin' oot on their puff likes"*. In other words, arthritis is bad enough in later life (puff), imagine developing it when you are in your twenties, your teens or even being born with this serious, painful and enervating condition. Juvenile Idiopathic -of unknown cause - Arthritis (JIA) is a condition where at least one joint become inflamed for at least six weeks, in people who are less than 16 years old. JIA is not always painful but the affected joints become stiff, swollen, warm to the touch and so mobility and movement are impaired. The whole series of conditions that are referred to as JIA are auto-immune diseases, the essential difference being that JIA affects those individuals who are less than 16 years old. As with its adult form JIA causes inflammation of the joints and supporting tissues.

JIA is the most common form childhood arthritis, affecting approximately 300,000 children in the US alone. The impact ranges from mild inflammation lasting a few weeks to major joint impairment which lasts into adulthood. In the most extreme cases, JIA leads to a complete collapse of the joint and supporting structures. Unfortunately for the female of the species the probability of developing JIA is about four times greater than for the male, particularly in the second decade of life. According to the UK National Rheumatoid Arthritis Society (NRAS), approximately 12,000 children are diagnosed (The NHS assets 15,000 children) with JIA making it one of the most common forms of physical disability in the country. The disease can manifest itself at any age from birth to 16 but 6 years old appears to be the peak onset year. Overall JIA is an autoimmune condition as discussed in both the *"crushing arthritis"* and *"crushing diabetes"* books. Hence at this juncture, it seems timely to remind the reader that a diet which contains foods that are linked inflammation must be avoided. In JIA the synovial (lubricating) fluid and connective tissue (cartilage) which enable the joints to function are targeted by the immune system of the child who develops it. In terms of its development and progression, JIA can be equated to the onset of adult forms such as rheumatoid arthritis and Osteoarthritis. JIA is comparable to its adult counterparts in terms of the damage it can cause to the musculoskeletal system and so is an equally undesirable disease.

As a disease JIA is broadly split into three forms, the first, oligo - (from the Latin for few) - articular JIA is the most common, affecting about 50% of all UK sufferers. Oligo-articular JIA develops from ages five and younger and affects less than four joints. For reasons that are unclear this form of JIA tends to affect the knee and ankle joints. One indicator of the disease is the inflammation of the eyes and a child blood test which reveals the presence of anti-nuclear antibodies (ANA's) is a recognised marker for this form of JIA. The conventional treatment involves corticosteroids which often have side effects and there is no guarantee that the steroids will be effective. In addition, remission can take several years to achieve, which is a crucial point to consider from a dietary perspective because oligo-articular JIA can lead to long lasting and / or permanent damage to the musculoskeletal system. Furthermore, one consequence of JIA is a simultaneous reduction in red blood cell count, (which can lead to symptoms of anaemia) and increased rates of blood sedimentation. The latter symptom is also considered a likely indicator of progression to polyarticular JIA.

As the term poly suggests, this form of JIA affects more than four joints and accounts for some 20% of all UK sufferers and has an affinity for the joints and tendons of the hands and feet. Polyarticular JIA is painful and sufferers often endure the additional trauma of secondary fevers when the disease "flares up". Conventional treatment involves Non-Steroidal Anti-inflammatory Drugs (NSAIDS) or immunosuppressive drugs which may well prevent joint damage but both classes of pharmaceutical are known to elicit side effects. Polyarticular JIA is a long-term and recurrent condition and is much more aggressive than oligoarticular JIA. Systemic onset JIA is identical to the polyarticular form but induces fevers which exceed 40°C which last for up to two weeks, rashes and causes swelling of the lymph nodes. Systemic onset JIA affects about 10% of all sufferers and is treated with steroids and / or drugs such as methotrexate (an immune system suppressant), which often has equally problematic side-effects. Some young people will make a full recovery. The longer term consequences of this form of JIA are highly variable and tend affect teenage boys more than girls. The remaining 10% falls under the term Enthesitis-related JIA and is most common in teenage boys. It affects the movable (synovial joints) and the junctures where tendons connect to the bones. These broad definitions are further sub-divided because each form of arthritis has a different aetiology, none of which are fully understood. JIA in particular and arthritis, in general, is analogous to disease such as cancer in that the medical profession does not consider arthritis a single disease. Although there is no cure for JIA or arthritis, in general, the symptoms can be managed by a whole plethora of anti-inflammatory and other medications. However, the side effects can be wide-ranging, severe and include liver damage, mass gain and a proclivity to secondary infections. For some sufferers, such impacts are seen as almost as undesirable as the disease they are supposed to treat.

Hence if these drugs are being used as a part of treatment for the condition then it is essential that the input of a professional dietician is sought. In terms of diet and appetite many steroids actually increase the desire to eat, can increase blood pressure and promote the deposition of calcium ions (Ca^{2+}) onto the bones. So, for instance, the diet must be tweaked to limit the ingestion of sodium (Na^+) and potassium (K^+) ions (i.e. salt) but must be laden with vitamin C and calcium. Hence any PBD that is used to control JIA must be altered as to best prevent as much as possible flare-ups of JIA. Eating a PBD will not in itself cure or even definitely prevent a flare up of JIA; however, it is absolutely true that such a diet is essential for healthy physical, emotional, and cognitive development. As with its adult counterpart and from a dietary perspective the best way to manage JIA is to live as full a life as possible and consume those foods which are known to aid in the development of the musculoskeletal system and act as anti-inflammatories. As the *“SIRT FOOD and metabolism”* book makes clear, there is no secret to achieving this aim and as such it is entirely possible to reduce the incidence of flare-ups by moving away from processed foods and towards those which have the nutrients the body actually needs. In other words, the same general dietary advice that would be given to all of us can be applied to those young people who are experiencing JIA.

Appetite suppression is a common symptom of JIA and is caused either by a flare-up of the disease itself or as a consequence of medicinal side effects. Put simply, a flare up upsets the normal hormonal balance and action of chemical communication in the body. As such aside from any specific benefits pertaining to JIA obtaining all the nutrients necessary to ensure a healthy metabolism is beyond essential. We all feel *"off our food"* when we are ill but if a child has a flare-up which causes impaired and painful movement of the jaw muscles or the synovial joints of the wrists and fingers, then believe he or she is not going to feel like eating even their most favourite food. In a public or social situation, a child will need to feel supremely confident in even asking for help in carrying out any task or activity. I mean to say, imagine trying to pierce a juice carton with a straw or unscrew a lid, if you can't move your fingers! If the nutritional input is compromised then the child will likely become more vulnerable to secondary infections and in really serious cases JIA can actually inhibit their growth and physical development. Although it is not the whole picture the emotional well-being of the child is absolutely critical to preventing and managing JIA. As discussed in the *"crushing arthritis"* book Calcium is essential for healthy ossification. Dietary sources of calcium include kale, mustard, tofu, spinach, turnip greens. The intake of calcium is not compromised if you are following a balanced PBD. Vitamin D is also crucial for ossification and resorption of calcium and good food sources of this vitamin are soy milk and cereal grains. On a final note, it will be explained that the advent of GM soya is a further reason to monitor the nutrient quota of any PBD.

Chapter 6:
Diet Related Cancers

For our purposes and from the perspective of diet most of the research concerning cancer in those who adopt a PBD focuses on the incidence of breast and colorectal cancer. Hence unless otherwise stated these cancers will be the focus of this chapter. The *"crushing cancer"* Book presented the mortality figures for cancer and showed that by far the biggest cancer killer is breast cancer in women and Lung cancer in men. In terms of prevention lung cancer induced by smoking is still by far the biggest overall cause of premature death by cancer around the world. Hence, the single biggest preventative measure that any individual can take is to stop smoking, easier said than done (and believe me I know), but there we are, it cannot be put any more succinctly. According to researchers using the guidelines of the WHO an increased intake of fresh fruits and vegetables is probably going to reduce your risk of developing CVD irrespective of your age. In terms of cancer, the main dietary culprit across the board is colorectal cancer, which has the dubious honour of being the third most fatal cancer in the World. According to world cancer research, 1.4 million new cases of colorectal cancer are diagnosed every year and the organisation imparts that a significant percentage of these diagnoses are largely preventable. When we consider that approximately 700,000 people die every year from this form of cancer the impetus to ditch the burgers, processed and cured meats and get on the grains and nuts becomes even stronger. Furthermore, the greater the severity of any obesity the greater is the probability of cancer developing on other tissues and organs of the body. The *"crushing cancer"* set out the nutritional case for a PBD (or at the very least a diet which curtails red meat consumption). The same is true of those cancers associated with childhood. In addition Low-fat vegan diets particularly good for preventing the onset of cancers linked to insulin resistance (i.e. obesity and T2DB), breast, colon and even prostate cancer. However, the diet must contain sufficient amounts of vitamin D (which can be a problem irrespective of diet), as a deficiency is implicated in an increased risk of cancer.

In the western world, a PBD tends to contain more tofu and soy foods as compared to an omnivorous diet. Researchers have focused on the efficacy of compounds such as isoflavone and have established that the compound may well protect the body against the incidence of breast cancer in later life if consumed on a regular basis during childhood. Conversely, excessive digestion of dairy foods in childhood has been implicated in the onset of colorectal cancer in adults. Clearly, there are many variables which preclude the stating of a causative link, therefore, it is about risk as a function of metabolism. Biochemically soy foods including tofu are a rich source of isoflavones; other sources include plants such as red clover. Furthermore for those of you fielding the kind of myths mentioned in chapter two you can impart that isoflavones are not present in nutritionally beneficial quantities in animal foods. It is well established that eating foods which contain isoflavones could protect against breast cancer in later life. This assertion should also measure against the onset of colorectal cancer as a result of eating red meat and excessive amounts of dairy foods, in later life.

This writing has indicated that the more red meat a person eats the greater is their risk of developing colorectal and prostate cancer. In addition, a PBD contains more of the entirety of active compounds which are widely believed to elicit cancer protective effects. Furthermore, the *"crushing cancer and diabetes"* books discussed the direct correlation between obesity and the development of certain cancers. In other words, an argument for killing at least two dietary issues with one proverbial dietary stone once again presents itself. It would seem that nutritional research is indicating very strongly that because a PBD is associated with a lower BMI that the incidence of certain cancers is significantly reduced. Concurrently, the phytochemicals in a PBD have been demonstrated to produce synergistic (mutually enhancing) effects and so we can all expect research to reveal that eating food X which contains phytochemical Y may boost the efficacy of phytochemical A which is found in food B. However, it will likely be stressed to the maximum possible degree that the best way to benefit from any effect is to eat a well-balanced PBD. In young people and adults, the phytochemicals are widely believed to inhibit several carcinogenic processes at a molecular and cellular level. For example, they are known suppress cancer cell proliferation by reducing the degree of metastasis (cancer cell transport to secondary sites). Furthermore, phytochemicals are known to suppress the rate of Cancerous DNA (adduct formation) this is the collective set of the process by which carcinogens bond with DNA in the nucleus. DNA adduct formation is a principle step in the onset of full-blown cancer. In their entirety, the phytochemicals promote cell apoptosis (death), inhibit the efficacy of the enzymes implicated in carcinogenesis as well those process which promotes angiogenesis (blood vessel formation).

From a dietary perspective, different foods have different levels of different phytochemicals bound into their structure and they are bound in different ways. Hence food preparation is key and in the case of children that means talking to them about why (for example) they may have a raw carrot in their packed lunch box on Wednesday, but some leftover steamed broccoli in a coleslaw on Thursday. From a preventative perspective, leguminous vegetables are known to inhibit colorectal cancer but this may be in part due to the curtailment of eating red meat in particular as part of a PBD as opposed to any definite cancer-fighting abilities within the plant. Never the less study after study shows us that legume, fruit and another vegetable intake is directly associated with a reduction in the incidence of cancer across the board. It is far too early to state definitively that a particular diet will prevent a given cancer but without a doubt, the writing is on the wall. There are many questions still to answer and the variables concerning the onset of cancer (many of which we do not yet understand) preclude us from saying that a PBD will protect against cancer per se. Due to the nature of the collective of diseases that we term cancer, this may never happen, what can be said is that the cancer-inhibiting effects of certain chemicals contained within the foods which constitute a PBD may be demonstrated to be a quantifiable factor in preventing certain forms of the disease.

Chapter 7:
Preventing Childhood Obesity

Perhaps the clearest and apparent example of how diet can have negative health impacts is the huge prevalence of type 2 diabetes in young people. Clearly, the book *"crushing diabetes"* discussed in some detail the reasons for the global spike in the incidence of this almost totally preventable metabolic disease. That type-2 diabetes is so apparent in teenage populations across the world is in itself merely one damning indictment of the current food production and distribution system. According to the international diabetes federation (IDF), some 450,000 children have diabetes, with very roughly 90% of this figure being type2-diabetes. In addition approximately 70,000 new cases are diagnosed every year; again approximately 90% develop the largely preventable form. The single biggest driver to what is justifiably referred to as a preventable epidemic in young people is the massive and concurrent increase in childhood obesity levels. And yes it really is that simple! Having said that, we have seen throughout this series of books that the causes of obesity across the board are as complex as they are inter-related.

In essence, the same arguments toward preventing obesity and its most obvious bedfellow type-2 diabetes in adults can be applied to its onset in young people. An excellent jumping off point for discussing obesity and diabetes in children is to present one of the many the findings of the Diabetes Control and Complications Trial (DCCT). This 10 year (1983-1993) epidemiological study involved approximately 1500 volunteers and established that levels of blood glucose in young people were on average 1% higher as compared to adults. The young people involved in the study all underwent the appropriate treatment regimens as adult participants. In addition, all received higher doses of insulin in the treatment of Type-1 diabetes. In addition, it is well established that insulin levels are much higher during the teenage years as well as during the onset of puberty itself. For Children not affected by either form of diabetes insensitivity to the action of insulin is highest over the ages 12 to 14 but this insensitivity normalises by the late teenage years.

The root cause of insulin resistance in young people has been under investigation for several decades. One obvious candidate for such resistance is the huge hormonal change that occurs once puberty is reached and adolescence progresses. In short, a whole range of both growth and sex hormones are released which cause long-term changes in the physiology and physical characteristics which occur over a period of several years. Hence all dietary factors being equal, these hormones are prime candidates for inducing insulin resistance in young people. During the teenage years and in biochemical terms the metabolism of glucose is characterised by a decrease in the oxidation of glucose and an increase in the oxidation of fatty acids. The balance between the rates of oxidation of each class of substance was first demonstrated in the 1960's and is known as the Randle Cycle. In essence, this cycle quantifies the degree to which different tissues use either glucose or fatty acids as an energy source (respiration) for their metabolism. In healthy metabolism glucose as the simplest carbohydrate is used first, with the fatty acids only being used once supplies of glycogen begin to run down. This metabolism was referred to in some detail in the "*crushing diabetes*" book. During the teenage years, the increased levels of growth hormones are known to increase the tendency for the body to break down fatty acids (lipolysis) at the expense of glucose, resulting in a steady accumulation of glucose in the blood stream and a potential for glucose insensitivity (that is type-2 diabetes) to express itself. Diabetic research has established that the inactivity of insulin during puberty and adolescence can decrease by up to 50%. Clearly, then any factor which can be incorporated into potentially reversing such realities must be welcome and once again the most obvious and arguably easiest factor is diet. This series of books has plainly stated the correct dietary choices to make in the prevention of type-2 diabetes and the diseases associated with the condition.

The notion that a PBD is an ideal mechanism for ensuring weight loss and thus bringing the body back into metabolic balance is nothing new. For example, a paper published in 2006 collated findings from approximately 90 epidemiological (population) studies. In essence, this published review established that across age, gender, ethnicity and social class that vegetarians and vegans had a much lower BMI than those who ate a non-PBD diet. Such findings are further augmented by press releases from organisations such as the WHO. In essence, the review suggests very strongly that a PBD diet will rapidly reduce the BMI of an individual and concurrently reduce the incidence of CVD, high blood pressure, stroke, and obesity. In addition, it stands to reason that if the diet is low in refined sugars (whose excess is converted to fatty acids) and fats then less fat will be accumulated in the first instance. As was outlined in the *"crushing diabetes"* book it is these substances that are the primary drivers of insulin resistance in sufferers of type-two diabetes. Another way to look at this fact is to state that a PBD diet facilitates the *"burning off / aerobic respiration"* of extra calories because the less ingested food is converted to fat. Overall the primary scientific literature is replete with findings which continually demonstrate that those who eat a PBD have a lower BMI than individuals who do not.

Further detailed and holistic epidemiological studies carried out later in the 21st century draw similar conclusions. For instance, a study carried out in 2008 asserts that without doubt meat in general and processed meat, in particular, is a key driver to the onset of type-2 diabetes as compared to individuals who do not eat any meat foodstuffs. According to the researcher who carried out this 17-year study, omnivores are up to 75% more likely to develop diabetes than vegetarians. Overall people who consume a PBD diet are significantly less likely to develop type-2 diabetes than those people who do not. The exact reason is unclear but it is widely believed that the phytochemicals and other nutrients contained within plant foods simultaneously curtail insensitivity to insulin and promote its action in the metabolism. In addition, it must be remembered that type-2 diabetes is largely preventable and so as the BMI is reduced the need for medications to treat the symptoms of diabetes steadily decreases. Irrespective of the debates concerning the validity of a PBD as means of preventing or curing disease, that surely has to be a good outcome.

Concluding Remarks

Aside from the nutritional benefits the single biggest reason for adopting a PBD is that once established dietary habits extend into adult life. In terms of disease prevention if young people are eating too much processed and refined foods then they are likely to develop some degree of negative and preventable health condition. From that perspective alone explaining to our children and peers, the why of adopting a PBD is paramount. The disease preventing credential of adopting a PBD are clear and apparent if not scientifically proven, in short, the risk of developing a nutritional disease is severely reduced. Having written that, without a doubt the debate concerning the virtues of A PBD will rage for the foreseeable future. A properly balanced PBD (based on fresh unprocessed ingredients) contains none of the saturated fats, extra calories, salt, sugar, additives that so characterise the western diet. In fact, because an organised PBD contains the entire nutrient needs of the body and is generally associated with healthier metabolism any potential concerns of nutrient deficiency can be resolved. Equally true are those research findings which inculcate that the risk of nutrient deficiency is higher in mothers who follow a PBD as compared to those who do not. This tells us once again that a person makes a choice as to whether to adopt a PBD and that pregnancy is probably not the best time to start experimenting with the diet. Furthermore, the point is made that education around food, nutrition and biological processes such as digestion is absolutely paramount irrespective of circumstances. Putting it directly a PBD means that a person has to take an interest in the biochemical process that convert the chemical energy contained within food into a form which drives metabolism and simultaneously releases chemicals which are believed to contribute to healthy physiology and disease prevention. If the reader is considering a PBD an overnight switch would not be advised, instead you should talk to friends, family and or professionals about what such a decision mean and arm yourself with the kind of knowledge discussed in these books. Furthermore, the food police are not going to come knocking on your door if you treat yourself to an old favourite occasionally. Speaking personally, If I was conversing with you about why the scientific evidence for climate change is so compelling I would expect you take the knowledge on board and at the very least think about it and engage with the issue by signing petitions and joining or supporting a campaign group on the issue. I have to practice what I preach and the science is telling me, more plants fewer animals and so I have to behave in an equivalent manner as far as my diet is concerned.

Sources

Primary Papers

http://www.thelancet.com/journals/lancet/article/PIIS0140-6736(13)60355-4/abstract

http://www.ncbi.nlm.nih.gov/pubmed/10687887

http://www.susanberkow.com/PDF/vegdietsandweightstatus3.pdf

http://www.nature.com/ejcn/journal/v61/n2/pdf/1602522a.pdf

http://enlivenarchive.org/2378-5438-1-2-004.pdf

http://www.ncbi.nlm.nih.gov/pmc/articles/PMC2812877/

http://ajcn.nutrition.org/content/89/5/1627S.full.pdf+html

http://www.ncbi.nlm.nih.gov/pmc/articles/PMC2391102/

http://ajcn.nutrition.org/content/86/6/1722.full.pdf

http://jn.nutrition.org/content/134/12/3479S.full.pdf+html

http://ajcn.nutrition.org/content/78/3/517S.full.pdf+html

http://carcin.oxfordjournals.org/content/14/10/2007.full.pdf+html

Books / Reviews

http://www.ncbi.nlm.nih.gov/pmc/articles/PMC3662288/

http://www.cps.ca/documents/position/vegetarian-diets

http://www.ncbi.nlm.nih.gov/pmc/articles/PMC4073139/

http://vegetarian.procon.org/sourcefiles/health_effects_of_vegetarian_and_vegan_diets.pdf

http://dge.stanford.edu/SCOPE/SCOPE_52/SCOPE_52_2.01_Beland_29-56.pdf

General sources

http://nutritionfacts.org/?s=plant+based+diets

http://www.who.int/mediacentre/factsheets/fs310/en/index2.html

http://www.who.int/mediacentre/news/releases/2014/child_mortality_estimates/en/

http://www.bbc.co.uk/news/health-21667065

http://www.pcrm.org/health/diets/vegdiets/vegetarian-diets-for-children-right-from-the-start

http://www.todaysdietitian.com/pdf/courses/PBDNutritentsofConcernPDF.pdf

http://www.nursingdegree.net/blog/19/57-health-benefits-of-going-vegan/

http://www.idf.org/global-idfispad-guideline-diabetes-childhood-and-adolescence

http://www.medscape.org/viewarticle/447138

http://healthyeating.sfgate.com/sources-isoflavones-8295.html

http://www.huffingtonpost.com/dr-mark-hyman/is-there-a-cure-for-autoi_b_756937.html

http://www.pcrm.org/health/diets/vegdiets/vegetarian-diets-for-children-right-from-the-start

Before you go

Thank you for purchasing my book!

If you found this book interesting and enjoyed reading it, I would really appreciate a short **review on Amazon**. All of your feedback is valuable to me, as your comments and input will be taken on board to help me make this and future books even better.

I would love hearing what you have to say. Please leave me a helpful REVIEW on Amazon.

Other Books by VIDDA Publishing

THE MEDICINE ON YOUR PLATE Series

Understanding Disease, Prevention & The Importance of Plant Based Nutrition and Diet

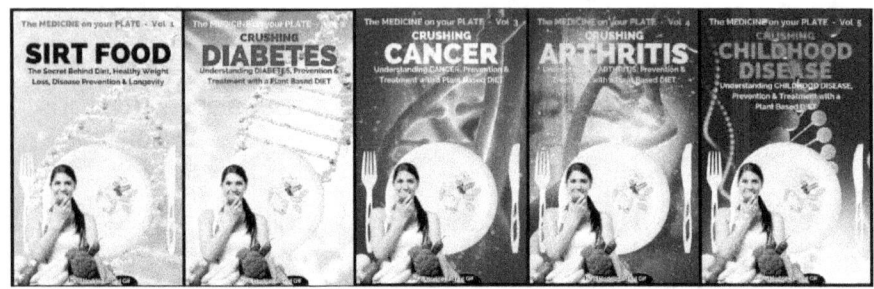

GREEN UP YOUR LIFE Series
Take control of your health and well-being by introducing Natural, Eco-Friendly habits into your daily routine.

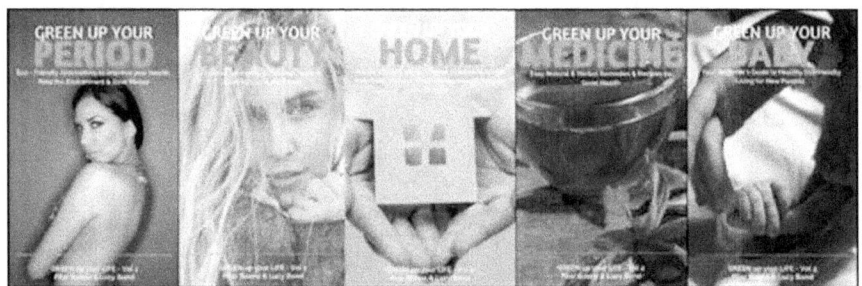

DOG TALES Series
Stories of Loyalty, Heroism & Devotion

BUSINESS, INCOME & SOCIAL MEDIA Series
How to Promote, Market & Create Business with Social Media

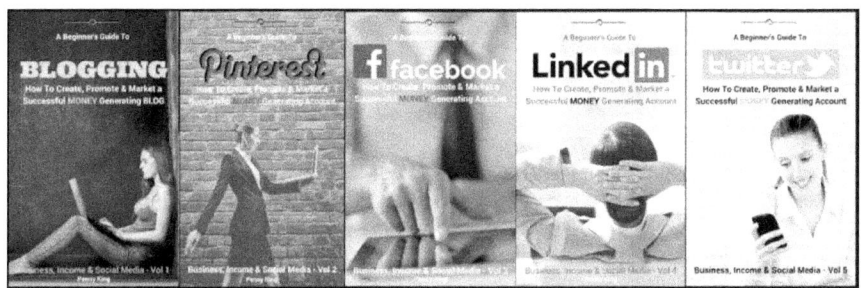

RESOLUTION TO BE HAPPY
Make yourself smile every day and banish stress and anxiety forever

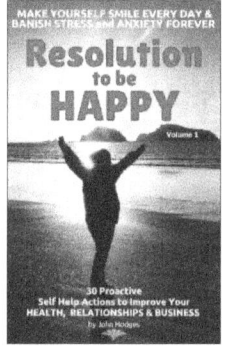

INTRODUCING GENETICALLY MODIFIED ORGANISMS - GMO
The History, Research, and The TRUTH You're Not Being Told

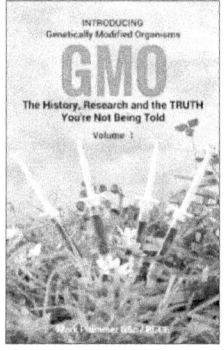

NATURAL WILD WINES

A Guide To Making Delicious Home Made Wine. Tips, Equipment, Recipes & Foraging Wild Fruits, Flowers & Herbs

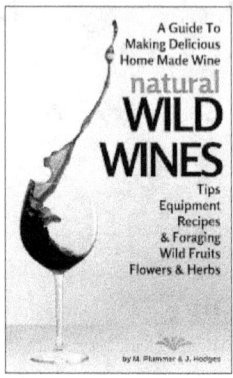

www.viddapublishing.com/books.html

Connect with John Hodges

If this book has helped you in any way or inspired you to take control of your own health and nutrition, it makes me a very happy man.

You can check out my publishing blog "Living Like You Mean It" (**viddapublishing.blogspot.co.uk**) for helpful tips, inspiration and updates on new books and free promotions coming soon.

You can also follow me on:

Twitter: twitter.com/VIDDAPublishing

John Hodges' Facebook: www.facebook.com/people/John-Hodges/550153788

VIDDA Publishing's Facebook: www.facebook.com/viddapublishing

For your Healthy, Nutritious, Green and Cruelty-Free products, equipment and gadgets, visit our online **VIDDA Health Stores** (US: **bit.ly/VIDDAstore** & UK: **bit.ly/VIDDAstoreUK**).

Also, for our favourite supplier of nutrients, sprouting seeds and health products, visit **bit.ly/BuyWholeFoodsOnline**

If you have any questions at all, please feel free to contact me at **viddapublishing.com/contact.html**

Wishing you the best of Health.

John Hodges

www.viddapublishing.com

www.themedicineonyourplate.com

www.sirtfood.com

www.greenupyourlife.org

www.ecologizatuvida.com